*To Sister Jeanette Haas: Your concern for others and quiet leadership
taught us the value of culture and inspired us to write this book.
Our sincere gratitude for all you have done.*

Leading Healthcare Cultures
How Human Capital Drives
Financial Performance

Your board, staff, or clients may also benefit from this book's insight. For more information on quantity discounts, contact the Health Administration Press Marketing Manager at (312) 424-9470.

This publication is intended to provide accurate and authoritative information in regard to the subject matter covered. It is sold, or otherwise provided, with the understanding that the publisher is not engaged in rendering professional services. If professional advice or other expert assistance is required, the services of a competent professional should be sought.

The statements and opinions contained in this book are strictly those of the author(s) and do not represent the official positions of the American College of Healthcare Executives or of the Foundation of the American College of Healthcare Executives.

Reprinted July 2017

Library of Congress Cataloging-in-Publication Data

Atchison, Thomas A., 1945–
    Leading healthcare cultures : how human capital drives financial performance / Tom Atchison and Greg Carlson.
        p. ; cm.
    Includes bibliographical references.
    ISBN 978-1-56793-303-1 (alk. paper)
    1. Health facilities—Personnel management. 2. Health facilities—Finance. 3. Corporate culture. I. Carlson, Greg (Gregory), 1953– II. Title.
    [DNLM: 1. Health Services Administration—economics—United States. 2. Organizational Culture—United States. 3. Health Facilities—economics—United States. 4. Health Facilities—organization & administration—United States. 5. Personnel Management—United States. W 84 AA1 A863L 2009]
    RA971.35.A83 2009
    362.11068'3—dc22
        2008041917

The paper used in this publication meets the minimum requirements of American National Standard for Information Sciences—Permanence of Paper for Printed Library Materials, ANSI Z39.48-1984. ⊚™

Acquisitions editor: Janet Davis; Project manager: Jane Calayag; Cover designer: Scott Miller

Health Administration Press
A division of the Foundation of the
   American College of Healthcare Executives
1 North Franklin Street, Suite 1700
Chicago, IL 60606-3529
(312) 424-2800

Introduction

If you want one year of prosperity, grow grain.
If you want ten years of prosperity, grow trees.
If you want a hundred years of prosperity, grow people.

—A Chinese proverb

The fact that the U.S. healthcare system is broken is no longer news to anybody. In this country, roughly 47 million people are uninsured (Medscape Today 2008) and medical errors continue to cause preventable deaths as well as to financially burden the system (*Washington Post* 2008). Since the Institute of Medicine (1999; 2001) published two landmark reports—*To Err Is Human* and *Crossing the Quality Chasm*—healthcare quality has become a national concern. National and international data indicate that the U.S. healthcare system will need to realize a 50 percent improvement to reach benchmark levels in outcomes, quality, access, and efficiency. Also, studies document that patients often do not receive proven therapies, that preventive measures are underutilized, and that the rates of preventable errors are unacceptably high (Schoen et al. 2006; McGlynn 1997; Schuster, McGlynn, and Brook 1998; McGlynn et al. 2003).

What's news to many, including healthcare leaders, is that the status quo has repeatedly failed us and much needs to be done to reverse the industry's downward spiral and help us navigate its landscape. Now is the time to make a dramatic change. (See Sidebar A for a historic perspective on change.) ▶

Healthcare leaders have the responsibility to initiate, participate in, and embrace change. Even this is not enough, however. Leaders must first learn to view change as a move toward progress, not as a response to failure, and they must engender this same attitude within their own organizational cultures. Those who become innovators and early adopters will increase their profitability and market share as well as their clinical quality, patient satisfaction, and employee satisfaction. Ideally, the improvements that take place inside hospitals, clinics, nursing homes, and other healthcare facilities will spread out to the wider field of care delivery and inspire better practices and policies.

SUSTAINABLE CHANGE

The first step to finding a solution is recognizing that a problem exists.

Consider an organization that is performing better financially than its competitors but is unconcerned about quality. Great financial performance is impressive, but financial excellence is only one dimension of success and does not factor in the satisfaction of the patient, the appropriateness of care, and the quality of care. Financial prosperity will be only temporary if healthcare providers do not ad-

dress the underlying problems that plague a healthcare system that has been characterized as "fragmented, inefficient, and expensive . . . [and] that neglects those who cannot pay, is deficient in defining and delivering quality services, and furthermore responds more to the financial interests of investors, managers, and employers than to the medical needs of patients" (IOM 2001).

SIDEBAR A

On January 31, 1829, Martin Van Buren, then governor of New York, sent the following letter to President Andrew Jackson.

Dear President Jackson,
The canal system of this country is being threatened by the spread of a new form of transportation known as "railroads." The federal government must preserve the canals for the following reasons:

One: If canal boats are supplanted by "railroads," serious unemployment will result. . . . Captains, cooks, drivers, hostlers, repairmen, and lock tenders will be left without means of livelihood, not to mention the numerous farmers now employed in growing hay for horses.

Two: Boat builders would suffer; towline, whip and harness makers would be left destitute.

Three: Canal boats are absolutely essential to the defense of the United States. In the event of the expected trouble with England, the Erie Canal would be the only means by which we could ever move the supplies so vital to waging a modern war.

As you may well know, Mr. President, "railroad" carriages are pulled at the enormous speed of 15 miles per hour by "engines" which, in addition to endangering life and limb of passengers, roar and snort their way through the countryside, setting fire to crops, scaring the livestock, and frightening the women and children. . . . The Almighty never intended that people should travel at such breakneck speed.

Respectfully,
Martin Van Buren

Source: Zenger-Miller (1987).

The longer we, as part of the healthcare industry, defer making needed changes, the more drastic the changes will need to be. That said, however, acting soon should not be mistaken for acting carelessly. Changes have to be strategic to yield sustainable results. This means that the interests of all our stakeholders (physicians, employees, insurance companies and other payers, and patients) must be aligned and that our focus must be on providing clinically appropriate, high-quality, and cost-effective care. To achieve alignment, we must seek out and understand the trends that influence our stakeholders and our practices. (See Sidebar B for an example of one of these trends.)

Sustainable changes, strategies, and success *cannot* occur within a dysfunctional culture. Healthcare organizations need to develop cultures that value human capital in the same way that financial capital is valued. A balanced commitment to both resources is necessary to achieve sustainable improvements within the organization and throughout the broader healthcare industry.

How do we get there? This book offers some guidance.

ABOUT THIS BOOK

The ideas in this book evolved over time from discussions among our colleagues about the factors that contribute to an organization's long-term performance and ultimate

---

SIDEBAR B

Beyond the walls of our hospitals and doctor's offices are a growing number of people who are leaving the United States to receive healthcare in foreign countries. These "medical tourists" were initially attracted to shop around for more affordable options outside of the U.S. healthcare system. However, many have had such a positive experience that their initial fears about the care quality abroad have dissipated. Although currently a silent minority, these medical tourists are sending a powerful message. Are we listening?

The cost of a surgical procedure in India, Thailand, or South Africa is approximately one-tenth the price (or sometimes cheaper) of the same service in the United States or Western Europe. For example, a heart-valve replacement that costs $200,000 or more in the United States is about $10,000 in India; this $10,000 includes the cost of the round-trip airfare and a brief recuperation/vacation package for the patient and a significant other. Similarly, a metal-free dental bridge that costs $5,500 here is priced at $500 in India. Lasik eye surgery that is worth $3,700 in America is available in many other countries for only $730. Cosmetic surgery savings are even greater: A full facelift priced at $20,000 in the United States costs about $1,250 in South Africa.

Although these savings sound attractive, many U.S. residents, except for "innovators and early adopters," believe that going overseas for healthcare services is too risky. Concerns about inferior medical care persist, and some skeptics believe that "third-world surgery" cannot possibly be as good as the care available in the United States. In fact, cases of botched plastic surgery have been reported, particularly from Mexican clinics. However, the Institute of Medicine's 1999 landmark report *To Err Is Human* has documented that poor care knows no geographic boundary. Overcoming incidents of errors is a growing pain for virtually all service industries and innovative companies.

The reality is that foreign hospitals and clinics that cater to medical tourists are some of the best in the world, with many staffed by physicians and caregivers trained at major medical centers in the United States and Europe. Another reality is that medical tourists seek out the best providers at the best price, and this practice is easier in today's global economy, where quality and cost of products and services are becoming more transparent.

Providers who protest against consumer scorecards or who try to retain market share by criticizing their competition (domestic and foreign) are fighting a losing battle. The only formula for success in a global economy is to produce the best product at the best price.

success. Certainly, financial capital is critical, as it allows organizations to operate their facilities, invest in equipment and technology, comply with various regulations, hire and retain staff, grow their business, and invest in research and development for the future. Equally important to an organization's long-term success is the development and retention of human capital. Successful organizations outperform their peers at recruiting, retaining, and developing their human resources.

After discussing and sharing our collective experiences, we arrived at our position that financial capital and human capital are equally critical to long-term success. However, the way each resource is managed, and subsequently thrives or dies, depends on the organization's culture. Organizational *culture* is the independent variable that separates the best organizations from average- and poor-performing organizations.

This book focuses on the interrelationships that exist between human resources and financial capital and their effect on the culture. Our experience and review of the literature have shown us that, traditionally, financial performance and human capital are viewed and addressed as separate and unrelated concepts. The reality, however, is that when organizations pay equal attention to both areas, they position themselves to outperform their competition. In this book, we enumerate how to achieve this balance.

CHAPTER CONTENTS

Chapter 1 explores organizational culture, the most critical component of any change process and the ultimate determinant of success. Institutions that have positive and participative cultures realize returns on investments that are nearly twice as high as organizations with less efficient cultures.

Chapter 2 discusses the role that finance plays in supporting the organization's culture. Finance and the finance team should be viewed as partners in building and maintaining a values-based culture that does its work to fulfill the organization's mission. In this chapter, we offer eight rules for ensuring that finance goes beyond its monetary focus to achieve long-term financial viability.

Chapter 3 presents the perspective that human capital is an organization's biggest investment. As such, employee issues should receive as much attention as is paid to financial issues. This discussion includes methods of developing, measuring, and understanding employee performance, satisfaction, and behavior. An organization's culture is only as strong as its people—that is a fundamental rule leaders must understand.

Each chapter submits some questions for leaders to ponder.

CONCLUSION

The current state of the U.S. healthcare system has ushered in more competition and mergers, reductions in reimbursement, ongoing workforce shortages, and the growth of medical tourism. These trends make it even more important for us to enhance our organizational culture, not only to carry us through the present but to sustain us into the future. We hope this book solidifies our argument.

REFERENCES

Institute of Medicine (IOM). 1999. *To Err Is Human.* Washington, DC: National Academies Press.

———. 2001. *Crossing the Quality Chasm.* Washington, DC: National Academies Press.

McGlynn, E. A. 1997. "Six Challenges in Measuring the Quality of Health Care." *Health Affairs* 16 (3): 7–21.

McGlynn, E. A., S. M. Asch, J. Adams, J. Keesey, J. Hicks, A. DeCristofaro, and E. A. Kerr. 2003. "The Quality of Health Care Delivered to Adults in the United States." *New England Journal of Medicine* 348 (26): 2635–45.

Medscape Today. 2008. "Census Bureau: Number of U.S. Uninsured Rises to 47 Million Americans Uninsured: Almost 5 Percent Increase Since 2005." [Online article; retrieved 7/23/08.] www.medscape.com/viewarticle/567737.

Schoen, C., K. Davis, S. How, and S. Schoenbaum. 2006. "US Health System Performance: A National Scorecard." *Health Affairs* 25 (6): w457–75.

Schuster, M., E. A. McGlynn, and R. H. Brook. 1998. "How Good Is the Quality of Health Care in the United States?" *The Milbank Quarterly* 76 (4): 517–63.

Washington Post. 2008. "Medical Errors Costing U.S. Billions." [Online article; retrieved 7/23/08.] www.washingtonpost.com/wpdyn/content/article/2008/04/08/AR2008040800957.html.

Zenger-Miller. 1987. *Dealing with Change.* Tampa, FL: Zenger-Miller, Inc.

CHAPTER 1

Culture Matters

Corporate culture . . . represents the taken-for-granted and shared assumptions that people make about how work is to be done and evaluated and how employees relate to one another and to significant others.

—Cummings and Worley (2004)

Culture is an organization's personality. It reflects the institution's established values and beliefs, and it dictates the attitudes, decisions, behaviors, responses, and interactions of every member of the organization. Because culture is created and maintained by the very people who inhabit it, no two corporate cultures are exactly alike. Each culture has its own set of rules and standards based on the mission, vision, and values of its host entity.

A culture is neither good nor bad. In fact, characterizing a particular culture as either good or bad is unfair, given that high performance is possible even within a "bad" culture ▶

and that mistakes occur even within a "good" culture. However, there is such a thing as a strong or positive culture.

A strong culture is carefully constructed by a team of skilled and dedicated leaders who believe the mission, support the vision, and live the values. In such a culture, organizational behaviors and values are aligned and human assets and financial capital are leveraged to achieve sustainable, long-term success.

In this chapter, we explore the many components of culture, providing sidebar examples and comments along the way.

THE FOUNDATION OF CULTURE

The mission, vision, and values articulate the basic function and philosophy of an organization. Creation, approval, and implementation of these three elements are the shared responsibility of the board of trustees and the CEO. All formal and informal leaders in the organization are expected to live the mission and clearly communicate the vision (as the saying goes, "leaders must constantly communicate the core values, and sometimes they may need to use words"). Furthermore, leaders must model behaviors that reflect established values. The mission, vision, and values shape, guide, and power the culture of an organization, just as the body, mind, and spirit do for the body.

The *mission statement* answers the following questions: "Why do we exist?" "Who are we?" "What do we do?" and "Whom do we serve?" In other words, the mission is a clear and brief expression of the organization's purpose. The *vision statement*, on the other hand, responds to these questions: "Where are we headed?" "Where do we want to be?" Simply, the vision is a declaration of the organization's dreams about what is possible, not probable, in the future.

Values are an organization's decision rules, beliefs, and moral compass, laying out the behavioral expectations for all the stakeholders in the institution—leaders, managers, physicians, clinicians, caregivers, and support staff. Values do not change over time, and they define the culture because they underpin all behaviors.

The culture influences all aspects of management and operations within an organization, including how leaders manage knowledge, encourage creativity, engage employees, and support the organization's philosophy about education and development (Baker 2007).

THE POWER OF THE VISION

As seen in Figure 1.1, strategies, tactics, and performance flow from the vision. A well-developed vision (which includes measurable goals) can inspire ideas, practices, and behaviors that enhance the capability of the organization to meet and exceed its goals. (See Sidebar C for an example of an inspiring vision.)

When individuals understand how their behaviors contribute to or detract from achieving the vision, they perform accordingly. This understanding is a seed to a shared value. For example, if employees are aware that tardiness not only creates

more work for everyone but also increases incidents of medical errors and causes patient and staff anxiety (all of which take away from the overall vision), then employees will not tolerate the behavior. As a result, timeliness becomes a shared value that permeates the culture.

Communicating the Vision

The chief leaders of the organization have the primary responsibility for educating all stakeholders regarding the following concepts:

1. What is the vision, and how is it linked to the mission and values?
2. What role does everyone play in achieving the vision?
3. How does an individual's behavior affect daily job performance and ultimately the success of the vision?

Leaders also have an obligation to inform stakeholders of their personal values, their philosophy of management, and their alignment with the core values. One of the best ways to communicate this information is by sharing life experiences related to the management or operational issue at hand. Illustrating professional points with personal stories is far more effective and memorable than

SIDEBAR C

In May 1961, President John F. Kennedy presented a bold challenge to the joint session of the U.S. Congress: Send a man to the moon by the end of that decade. Some people derided this dream as lunacy, while others viewed it as just another strategic move in the Cold War chess match between the United States and the Soviet Union. JFK's vision had a clear timeline of under ten years. Most importantly, this vision was inspirational, moving thousands of people to craft a careful and effective strategy and to change their behavior to accomplish the goal.

Figure 1.1. Elements of Vision

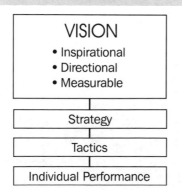

VISION
- Inspirational
- Directional
- Measurable

Strategy

Tactics

Individual Performance

regurgitating formal policies and statements.

Clear and constant communication leads to understanding, and understanding ultimately results in commitment, which is a critical contributor to the success of any undertaking. Leaders who are not aware of this dynamic typically make tactical, not strategic, decisions; tactical steps are appropriate primarily on a departmental level. Individuals need communication to understand how their specific work and behavior contribute to achieving the overall mission and vision. Without this clear framework, people default to a "what is best for me" mind-set, which is a clear path to failure.

Communication also enables or reinforces a culture of inclusion. The implicit message behind any communication should be an invitation to participate, whether by commenting on the information or by getting involved in a project or decision. When leaders seek input from the organization's stakeholders (who by the nature of their jobs are the experts in their field), the effect is powerful. Not only do employees become more committed, but they also feel a stronger connection with the organization and with their colleagues.

VALUES-BASED CULTURE

Values not only support the accomplishment of the vision but also define the culture. Created and reinforced by years of practice, values are expressed through the words and behaviors of the individuals in the organization as they perform their daily activities. For example, a culture's customer service orientation or values may be manifested in the way the receptionists make eye contact when they greet visitors, or when a nurse offers a waiting family member something to read. These behaviors are driven by the values espoused by the culture. A culture is considered strong when the behaviors exhibited are values-based and are consistently exhibited throughout the organization (Atchison 2003).

More and more organizations are publishing their values on their website. This practice is intended to inform employees, customers, and the general public how the organization conducts itself in the course of carrying out its mission. Unfortunately, publicized values are often ignored or used only in marketing and promotional materials.

See Sidebar D for an example of a values-based culture.

Consistency

Organizational leaders must consistently model and communicate values-based behaviors, and they must consistently use values-based practices across the enterprise. Without this reinforcement, the culture atrophies and the return on human capital cannot be realized. The notion of overcommunicating the values of an organization—through newsletters, press releases, websites, and staff meetings, for example—should not be a concern when the ultimate goal is to achieve sustainable success. We have never heard of organizational problems that stemmed from overcommunicating expectations.

Consistency can be evaluated using two measures:

1. Are employee values, behaviors, programs, and practices consistently applied, regardless of department or manager?
2. Are organizational values and behaviors consistently reinforced, regardless of the organization's current performance?

The answers to these two questions should be a resounding "yes!" All efforts to build a strong culture will be for naught if the organization tolerates behaviors that are inappro-

priate, destructive, and not aligned with established values. This is true regardless of who is not modeling the values—the CEO, a physician, a nurse, or a transporter. Likewise, if leadership abandons the values when times are tough, employees will lose respect for management and will drop their support for the mission, vision, and values.

LONG-TERM OUTCOMES

Return on Investment

In 2003, the *Harvard Business Review* published the findings of a groundbreaking, five-year study that involved 160 companies. The report identified culture building as one of four management practices that produce superior results; the other three practices are talent management, leadership, and innovation. All of these practices are a reflection of a positive culture. According to the study, companies that mastered or followed these practices within a ten-year period consistently outperformed their industry peers: These companies realized a 95 percent return on investment (ROI), compared to the 62 percent ROI achieved by organizations that did not make the same commitment to culture (Nohria, Joyce, and Roberson 2003).

Recruitment and Retention

Culture is always the biggest determinant of employee satisfaction. The reason is that culture influences the types of employees (including physicians) recruited and retained. Simply stated, a strong culture has a direct effect on an organization's human capital.

VALUES ALIGNMENT. Organizations that hire, retain, and promote individuals whose personal values are aligned with the corporate values experience low turnover, high productivity, and improved employee and patient satisfaction. Conversely, organizations that do not seek or work toward alignment of values seldom realize the potential for superior performance, job satisfaction, and long tenure among their employees.

The basic assumption in values alignment is that values motivate individuals to support the vision and mission of the organization, making them more apt to contribute to achieving organizational goals. A strong culture reinforces the benefits of aligned values. As a result, organizations with strong cultures have employees who are committed, are productive, are innovative, and understand the value of teamwork. These predictable outcomes play a large role in achieving sustainable success.

COMPETENCY. Another focus of a strong culture is to recruit and retain the most competent individuals available. A practice of promoting from within makes this goal easier to accomplish, given that many times the desired talent and expertise (not to mention the aligned values) already exist amid the current staff pool. (See Sidebar E for an example of a successful application of values alignment and promotion from within.) In a strong culture, promoting from within is usually possible because its leaders encourage

The following cases focus on an organization with a values-based culture. Both cases illustrate that values have to be ingrained in daily practices and policies for them to make an impact.

Case 1

Shortly after accepting the chief operating officer position at Main Community Hospital, Alicia Lopez was thrust into the newly vacant CEO role. As the newly appointed CEO, Lopez was faced with an immediate challenge: to transform the performance of the surgery department, where the manager turnover was high and the staff attitude was becoming increasingly negative.

Lopez was a new CEO, but she was not new to the organization itself. She had worked her way up from a staff nurse role. She understood the culture of the hospital, and she was grateful that one of its deeply held values was to retain high-performing employees through continuous education and training and internal promotion. For more than 20 years, Lopez has lived these values.

After hearing the problems with the surgery department, Lopez privately consulted with three respected members of the medical staff, each of whom recommended that Vicki Richards, known as the "best manager in the hospital," be brought in to head the surgery department. Lopez had heard of Richards's good reputation and great work in the ICU. Richards was an ICU nurse, not a manager, but she had constantly provided management help when needed. Lopez thought it was time that Richards was promoted, so she immediately approached her for the management position in the surgery department. However, Richards politely said no, citing love for her post at the ICU and her inexperience with the surgical team. Lopez insisted, and Richards reluctantly agreed.

At her first meeting with the department staff, Richards laid out the organization's values; her values and expectations; and her plan to improve the service, quality, and relationships in the department. She instituted new processes and policies that put the values into action; that were more efficient; and that focused on enhancing patient, employee, and staff satisfaction. She modeled behavior that demonstrated her fairness and her concerns for everyone. Although most staff embraced this new approach, some employees did leave.

Several months later, the surgery department began to show signs of improvement. Employee attitudes were changing, and physicians were being more cooperative. More time passed, and better results were evident. The hospital's best nurses, technicians, and other support staff and caregivers were clamoring for an opportunity to work in surgery. Physician referrals were rising, care outcomes were measurably improved, and incidents of medical errors were decreasing.

Case 2

In another part of Main Community Hospital, Lopez began to hear disgruntled rumblings through the grapevine about the finance department. The topic of ire was Guy Barthes, the newly hired director of reimbursement at the department. According to staff, Barthes was impossible to work with. He was rude, inflexible, and unfair to his direct reports. He penalized staff for not following established processes and policies, but he regularly broke them for his benefit. He did not offer training, coaching, and advocacy for his employees, but he expected perfect performance at all times. Although he had only been employed at the hospital for one year, Barthes should have been aware that his disruptive behavior could not be tolerated in a values-based culture.

Lopez discussed these concerns with the vice president of finance, who promised to investigate the matter and to take appropriate action. After a thorough investigation and numerous discussions with Barthes about the issue (even providing him with a crash course in the mission, vision, and values and a chance to correct his ways), the vice president had no choice but to terminate Barthes.

This termination inspired a lot of awe among staff, many of whom claimed, "They are really serious about this culture stuff."

ongoing training, continuing education, and professional development.

When recruiting from outside the organization, the most effective strategy to ensure values alignment is to construct job descriptions that incorporate the established values. Such a description serves as a guideline for evaluating the fit of an outside candidate, and it also may be used to assess internal applicants. If any human resources function (recruitment, retention, selection, evaluation, promotion) steers away from these stated values, the values shrink in importance, which in turn invites self-interests and other dysfunctional personal motivations.

EMPLOYEE SATISFACTION. Herzberg (2003) conducted a review of 12 separate studies to identify the factors that affect employee attitudes and lead to extreme job satisfaction or dissatisfaction. According to Herzberg, the three highest-ranking motivators of job satisfaction are (1) achievement, or having an opportunity to excel; (2) recognition, or being recognized for an accomplishment; and (3) the work itself, or being able to work on meaningful projects. On the other hand, the highest-ranking causes of job dissatisfaction are (1) company policies and administration, or too many rules; (2) supervision, or ineffective leadership; and (3) interpersonal relationships, or coworkers do not get along and staff behaviors are not guided by clear values.

The most striking observation from Herzberg's findings is that all motivators and causes of dissatisfaction are directly related to organizational culture. Interestingly, pay was not mentioned on either list. Our collective experience suggests that pay becomes a major issue only when an organization does not provide the "intangibles"—factors such as worthwhile work and development opportunities. Pay, in this scenario, becomes a tangible reason for leaving.

THE ROLE OF TRUST

Trust is the glue that holds a culture together; it is also the lubricant that reduces friction during stressful times. Without trust, the organization's mission, vision, and values are mere jargon, creating an illusion of success. With trust as a basis of everyone's interaction, the culture is strengthened, allowing everyone in the organization to work toward the mission, vision, and values (see Figure 1.2).

Figure 1.2. Strength of Trust

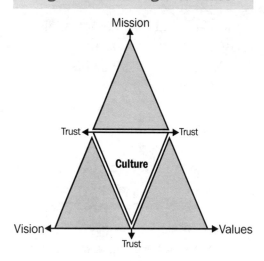

Trust is an outcome; it is not something we do. It is a product of a person's conscious effort and commitment to be open, honest, and consistent. As such, it is within a person's control. The frequency of meaningful interactions increases trust, and frequency and meaningful interactions can be controlled by the individual. For example, in an effort to build trust, a CEO can regularly spend time talking (formally or informally) with frontline staff. When conducted with sincerity and truthfulness, such dialogues over time will build trust between the two parties.

Perception is critical in trust. For example, when followers (employees) observe that their leaders (executives and managers) tell the truth, share relevant information, and behave predictably, they are more likely to trust these leaders. "Liking" someone is not a requirement for trust. Liking and trusting are two separate dynamics; one is not a prerequisite for the other. Liking the person you trust is a bonus because it creates less tension in the relationship, but in the workplace, you do not have to like the person you trust.

Building Trust

Trust does not happen by accident. It requires an investment of time and effort, resources that are too often squandered on fixing day-to-day problems. Look at your schedule. How many minutes per day do you spend with physicians and other clinicians, managers, and support staff? What percentage of your daily interactions with these stakeholders involves trust building and strengthening?

MEANINGFUL INTERACTIONS. As mentioned earlier, meaningful interactions are the basis of trust. Listening fuels meaningful interactions, allowing the exchange between two parties to move forward. Successful leaders schedule agenda-free meetings with key physicians, community members, and staff to listen to their respective issues. By doing this, leaders can identify problems and solutions and show they care. Trust always results when people perceive that they have been heard or "truly listened to."

ACTIVE LISTENING. The type of listening proposed here is not the kind practiced in our society, where listening has become a lost or diminished art. True listening is not about waiting your turn to speak so that you can defend your points, nor is it about passively nodding your head to indicate your interest. The type of listening required in meaningful interactions is active listening.

The goal of active listening is to understand and learn rather than challenge and win. Active listening is a learned skill, and it begins with the suspension of predispositions, biases, and prejudices. In active listening, each party uses appropriate, refining questions to clarify points. This practice engenders trust and ensures that both parties understand the other's position or perspective.

For example, consider this interaction between a physician and a senior executive:

Physician: There's a lot of pressure in practicing medicine today.

Executive: Healthcare has changed. Get used to it.

With such a response, how do you think the physician will react?

That physician, from this point on, will not only distance himself from the executive but will also lose respect for this leader. The ultimate result will be that the executive destroys any possibility of alliance with the physician.

This type of scenario is not possible with active listening. Using active listening, the executive will offer the following responses: How have healthcare changes affected your practice? What can the hospital do to lessen the difficulties you face?

MAINTENANCE. In his seminal work, *The Fifth Discipline*, Peter Senge (1990) talks about the "trust bank account." This term relates to the need for leaders to continue to maintain and build trust, even (or especially) during conflict-free, low-pressure periods. Accumulating a lot of trust "savings" in this account helps leaders confront challenges in difficult times, given that trust acts as a lubricant in relationships—that is, trust eases the tension inherent in organizational interactions. When two people who trust each other disagree, the possibility of an ideal outcome is high. Thus, maintaining trust is critical.

CHANGING THE CULTURE

Culture is the product of the organization's human capital. As such, it will change over the life cycle of the organization. Leaders need to recognize and accept this fact. According to Baker (2007), successful companies cannot continue to excel if they do not change. In fact, a key attribute of high-performing organizations is a culture that can change and adjust according to its internal and external environments and needs (Collins 2001).

Changing the culture involves three steps (Heathfield 2008):

1. understanding why change is needed,
2. creating a vision for the future that spells out how the change will be accomplished, and
3. having a commitment to change behaviors to fit the desired culture.

Cultures develop over many years and remain in effect for many gener-

ations, so introducing a new culture is a tremendous feat. Such change is typically difficult and slow (Heathfield 2008). However, organizations can learn a lot from the past while they develop a new focus for the future.

QUESTIONS FOR LEADERS

1. Have your organizational values been converted to behaviors that enhance human resources, trustee, and medical/clinical decisions, among others?
2. Can each of your strategic imperatives be connected directly to the organization's mission, vision, and values?
3. How much time do the board of trustees and the CEO invest in learning about better ways to use the mission, vision, and values in decision making?
4. Do you schedule time (at least 60 minutes per day) for building trust with individuals who are critical to the organization's success?

REFERENCES

Atchison, T. 2003. *Followership*. Chicago: Health Administration Press.

Baker, J. 2007. Personal communication with the authors.

Collins, J. 2001. *Good to Great: Why Some Companies Make the Leap . . . and Others Don't*. New York: HarperBusiness.

Cummings, T. G., and C. G. Worley. 2004. *Organization Development and Change*, 8th ed. Florence, KY: South-Western College Publishing.

Dadlez, C. 2007. Personal communication with the authors.

Heathfield, S. 2008. "How to Change Your Culture: Organizational Culture Change." [Online information; retrieved 7/3/08.] www.about.com.

Herzberg, F. 2003. "One More Time: How Do You Motivate Employees?" *Harvard Business Review* 81 (1): 87–96.

Nohria, N., W. Joyce, and B. Roberson. 2003. "What Really Works." *Harvard Business Review* 81 (7): 42–52.

Senge, P. 1990. *The Fifth Discipline*. New York: Doubleday Business.

CHAPTER 2

Eight Rules for
Managing
Finance in a
Values-Based Culture

Incorporating the finance team in daily operations can provide a number of benefits.

Sustainable financial performance begins with a values-based culture. As explained in Chapter 1, organizational values serve as a compass for behaviors. The values must be communicated to employees, physicians, and leaders to clarify the organization's philosophy and expected behaviors. Failure to do so will result in misalignment of values, which leads to organizational dysfunction. The key to long-term success is the values alignment within and between units, departments, and groups. For example, the finance department cannot play by a set of rules or values that conflicts with ▶

or differs from the rules followed by the medical staff and the rest of the organization.

Based on our observation, the finance department is often not fully integrated into the culture of an organization. Managers, directors, and vice presidents often view members of the financial team as "bean counters" or "cost cutters" whose main reason for existence is to withhold or restrict funds and resources. This mind-set undermines the value of teamwork, a critical building block of a strong culture. The budgeting process is more stressful, more time consuming, and less efficient when members of the financial team are not viewed as partners.

The eight rules in this chapter are intended to transform the way the finance department is viewed, providing an explanation of how finance functions within a healthcare organization. Organizations that follow these rules put themselves in a greater position to strengthen their culture and to leverage the talents and expertise of their financial team as a partner in their mission-fulfilling work.

Because finance is the language of business, all healthcare leaders and managers are more effective when they understand basic financial concepts and terminology. Incorporating the finance team in daily operations provides a number of benefits, such as an exchange of knowledge between the finance department and the rest of the staff (including physicians); a less contentious budgeting process; an improvement in financial decision making; greater alignment between the clinical staff and the finance team, with a focus on the mission, vision, and values; and better financial performance.

RULE 1: INVOLVE THE MEDICAL STAFF

The business model for hospitals is unique among U.S. companies. In no other industry are organizations (hospitals) so dependent on a group of individuals (physicians) who are often not their employees and who are sometimes their competitors. Hospitals provide physicians a "workshop" in which to practice their profession and treat patients, but physicians are typically not employed by the hospital, which pays for the facilities, the equipment, and the support staff (Berenson, Ginsburg, and May 2006). Physicians must apply for *privileges* to treat patients at the hospital, which also allow them to bill (separately from the hospital) for the services they provide.

In the past, physicians and hospitals had a relationship that was collaborative and cooperative. Seldom, if ever, did hospitals and physicians compete with each other. A culture of mutual support existed, where physicians served on committees and took calls to ensure the hospital had the ability to respond to the needs of patients, whether they could pay or not. The business model for both physicians and hospitals was based on a cross-subsidized pricing structure, in which some patients were charged higher rates to make up for losses incurred in treating those without health insurance or the ability to pay. A by-product of this system was a lack of price transparency that kept insured patients unaware of, or insulated from, the true cost of services (Burns, Anderson, and Shortell 1993).

Managed care, increased competition, rising costs, and reductions in reimbursement have transformed this culture of collaboration between hospitals and physicians into a culture of competition. Today, many physicians refuse to take calls; demand payment to serve on hospital committees; and compete directly with hospitals for the most profitable services, such as lab and ancillary services. In many communities physicians own free-standing surgery centers, and, in a limited number of states, physicians have built and operate specialty hospitals.

Of all the factors that contribute to higher-quality outcomes and lower costs, the degree of alignment between physicians and hospitals is critical. Alignment occurs when organized delivery systems share the same mission, vision, goals, objectives, and strategies. Shortell and colleagues (2001) argue that collaboration results in improved quality and efficiency and ushers in better clinical and economic outcomes. The absence of alignment creates conflict, with both parties competing with each other and undermining the efforts of the other.

Two independent studies (Fisher et al. 2006; Shortell et al. 2001) documented improved performance and other benefits when hospitals and physicians coordinated their efforts and focused on common goals. One study detailed the efforts of a hospital and its medical staff to present themselves as a single locus of accountability; in doing so, both entities were evaluated together, instead of separately. This study aimed to determine if hospitals with a more tightly affiliated medical staff achieved higher performance than did hospitals without this type of relationship with its physicians (Fisher et al. 2006).

Continued deterioration of the relationship between physicians and hospitals has resulted in financial hardships for hospitals, forcing them to drastically cut expenses, eliminate services, and even go out of business (Altman, Shactman, and Eilat 2006). Clearly, this type of dysfunction has to change. Including physicians in efforts to establish or review the organization's values and mission can serve as a catalyst to enhancing hospital–physician relationships.

For more information on physician involvement, see Sidebar F.

Breaking Down Silos

One strategy for ushering in better hospital–physician relationships is for both parties to engage in constructive dialogue focused on creating an alignment of interests. Such an alignment benefits both parties and, more importantly, the patients they serve. The best place to begin is to tear down the organizational silos within hospitals and between the institution and its medical staff. Working as partners, hospitals and physicians can address the challenges facing the healthcare industry, including the fact that healthcare spending is growing at a much faster rate than the rest of the economy. Without fundamental changes, the majority of federal revenues (tax receipts) are estimated to go to healthcare between the years

---

SIDEBAR F

Historically, although hospitals and physicians did not compete against each other, they did not closely interact either. Administrators and boards of trustees rarely sought the input of the medical staff regarding strategic and management issues. Often, in-depth discussions between physicians and administrators occurred only after a problem surfaced. One consequence of this lack of consultation was that each party's strategies and objectives directly conflicted with one another. Today, hospitals and physicians do compete for the same business, but they still hardly communicate their interests and needs with each other. This practice must change.

Medicine and hospital administration are independent but highly interrelated disciplines. Administrators ensure the smooth operation of the hospital business, while physicians bring in much of that business. They dictate the type of treatment, services, and care setting. They can attract and refer patients. They can control clinical cost, quality, and outcomes. They are integral in achieving improvement goals. That said, no reasonable justifications can be made for excluding physician input in daily and strategic business and management decisions. A proactive effort to involve physicians can go a long way toward easing strained relations, dissuading direct competition, encouraging partnerships and support in all kinds of initiatives, controlling costs, reducing service duplication, promoting wellness and prevention rather than incentive-driven and costly interventions, and increasing physician satisfaction with the practice of medicine. These are achievable outcomes.

Healthcare leaders may solicit physician input with the following techniques:

- Routinely meet with formal and informal physician leaders to listen to their concerns and ideas.
- Periodically distribute a short survey to physicians that poses questions such as, "What is interfering with your ability to practice effectively?" and "How can the organization help you provide better care to patients?"
- Focus the discussions with physicians on the needs and wants of patients, not on the personal demands of physicians. According to a study by Berenson, Ginsburg, and May (2006), the level of physician satisfaction with medical practice in the United States is low. Physicians cited multiple dissatisfiers, including the limited time they can spend with patients and the lack of incentives for high-quality care. On the basis of these findings, it seems that much of the answer to "what makes physicians happy?" lies in giving them the opportunity to do a good job.

2016 and 2020 (Steuerle and Bovbjerg 2008).

Silos and self-interests develop when cross-departmental interactions do not occur on a regular basis. In this situation, employees and physicians are focused only on their own functional areas and do not have the knowledge, time, or skills necessary to connect with people outside of their own units. Silos limit or prevent interaction among financial personnel, other employees, and the medical staff. In 2002, the American Management Association published the results of a survey of 500 respondents. Eighty-three percent of respondents acknowledged the existence of silos within their organizations, and of these individuals, more than 90 percent viewed silos as a negative force in the culture and 7 percent considered them to be destructive (American Management Association 2002).

Breaking down silos is critical. Organizations without silos are transparent—that is, performance data are voluntarily shared throughout (and sometimes outside of) the organization. This transparency is a prerequisite to building trust. Our experience suggests that when members of the organization, regardless of their positions or expertise, work together, performance is enhanced. Teamwork is especially critical during periods of significant change, which characterize our current healthcare environment. Strategies for eliminating silos include the following:

- Hold regular meetings with employees and physicians from various (if not all) departments. This strategy creates an atmosphere of familiarity for staff and clinicians, many of whom normally may not venture out of their own units. After several meetings, relationships may develop and the seeds of trust may take root, which are two prerequisites for a positive culture (see Chapter 1).
- Create strategies that add value to the entire organization rather than strategies that benefit only one department.
- Seek participation and involvement from a wider mix of employees. Groups are generally better at solving complex, multifaceted problems than are individuals.
- Build or strengthen team orientation. Setting goals, monitoring outcomes, promoting cooperation, and sharing success are fundamental in a team-oriented culture (Nohria, Joyce, and Roberson 2003).

Improving Performance

A study by McKinsey & Company explored the drivers of productivity in industrial settings in the United Kingdom. The study covered 27 dimensions of management across four categories: Lean management, talent management, performance management, and leadership. For healthcare, McKinsey decided to test the hypothesis that direct involvement of doctors in the management of a hospital helps to improve the institution's performance. The study found that (1) a positive correlation exists between the level of physician involvement and hospital performance, and (2) physician input drives best practices (*McKinsey Quarterly* 2008).

RULE 2: INCORPORATE FINANCIAL EXPECTATIONS INTO ORGANIZATIONAL VALUES

Many not-for-profit organizations select "feel good" values—that is, those that appeal to emotions but are often impractical to follow. Other not-for-profits are hesitant, or even apologetic, to promote values related to finance for fear of compromising their charitable missions. Both practices are a mistake. Values must reflect the behaviors exhibited in the daily provision of services. Values are more about what is done than

what is said; this is true for organizations as well as for individuals.

Failure to incorporate finance-related expectations into organizational values sends the implicit message that financial performance is not important. Articulating the value of finance serves to foster and enhance relationships between members of the financial staff and staff in other departments. In organizations with values-based cultures, members of the financial team have regular interactions with all departments and all groups, including the medical staff. Such a working relationship not only broadens the financial staff's understanding of the care-giving function, but it also encourages the financial staff to become advocates for the goals and needs of different units. The practice of inclusion creates a culture of teamwork, participation, and involvement, where employees and physicians develop a sense of ownership and a sense of belonging.

RULE 3: EDUCATE MANAGERS ON THE BASICS OF FINANCE

Healthcare managers, directors, vice presidents, and even some CEOs who began their careers as clinicians view finance as a foreign language, even a necessary evil in their new profession. This mind-set is common for those who trained and worked for years as clinicians before transitioning into management positions. Again, finance is the language of business, and as such, it is present in all enterprises, including the healthcare industry. New healthcare administrators, including physician executives and those who run their own practices, quickly realize that a fundamental knowledge of finance is required to become an effective manager.

Financial metrics and ratios are used to evaluate and compare performance. Managers who do not understand the key metrics and ratios used to analyze and compare their departments will have a difficult time making the adjustments necessary to operate their units and improve their performance. As mentioned in Chapter 1, organizations with strong, values-based cultures invest sufficient resources to educate and train employees in various fields and disciplines. In fact, providing top-of-the-line training and development programs is a retention strategy for these organizations (Nohria, Joyce, and Roberson 2003). Educating employees, particularly managers, on the basics of finance will yield a positive return on investment for any organization.

Five Functions

Finance performs five common functions. Knowledge of these functions allows managers to operate their respective service areas and to contribute to the financial goals and initiatives of the larger organization.

1. *Develop a budget and report actual performance compared to the budget.* Finance is responsible for recording the services rendered and their costs, the purchase or sale of assets, and the investment or borrowing of funds. Simply stated, a budget is a plan that anticipates and estimates the amount of resources needed to carry out the various activities of the business. As assumptions and events change, the budget also needs to change. For example, the cost of resources, such as pharmaceuticals, may have been budgeted at a certain price during a given time, but events in the overall economy will influence the decrease or increase of this budgeted cost. When this occurs, the budget needs to be adjusted. Using ratios to express the budget makes it easier to showcase how the unit or organization is performing over time and in comparison to its competition. A number

of resources can help familiarize nonfinancial managers with financial ratios, one of which is a publication by the Healthcare Financial Management Association (2007) titled *Key Hospital Financial Statistics and Ratio Medians*.

2. *Manage costs, increase revenue, and make the necessary adjustments to achieve the budget.* This task is done by analyzing the financial and statistical reports on all aspects of hospital operations. Use industry benchmarks to show managers if they are managing efficiently.

3. *Guard against theft, waste, and loss.* Management and the board must be assured that the organization's assets—both cash and noncash—are recorded, tracked, and accounted for in a secure manner.

4. *Assist management and the board in short-term and long-term planning.* Part of this function is to guide the organization through the budget process by advising and assessing the costs and financial risks of strategic alternatives. Budgeting is a matter of making choices about how and where to invest limited resources.

5. *Arrange funding for capital projects approved by governance.* This function should reflect the organization's philosophy on debt and its tolerance for risk. Decisions on short-term and long-term debt should take into account past performance, prospects for the future, and external factors that may influence short-term and long-term performance.

One strategy for educating staff about finance *and* promoting relationships (between the finance department and the rest of the institution) is to make members of the financial team available as teachers, or mentors, to clinical managers and physicians. As stated earlier, interaction between these two sets of professionals can lead to a greater appreciation for what the other does. The finance team is the most capable of educating the staff about budgeting, capital decision making, and all other financial functions.

RULE 4: VIEW THE FINANCE TEAM AS PARTNERS

Too often, the chief financial officer and the second-highest-ranking member of the financial team are the only ones represented on the management team. This practice is a holdover from organizational structures that reinforced silos, where clinical managers were expected to focus exclusively on clinical or caregiving matters while the finance department was assigned to deal solely with funds.

Organizations that seek to create strong cultures should look for opportunities for the finance team to become involved in strategic planning, operational activities, and committee work. This participation can be beneficial to the work carried out by physicians, other clinicians, and support staff. Partnership, collaboration, and regular interaction between departments facilitate the exchange of knowledge. While clinicians learn financial insights, the finance team carries away a better appreciation for day-to-day operations and challenges in healthcare delivery. Both sets of knowledge then inform budgeting and other financial decisions.

RULE 5: SET AND COMMUNICATE CLEAR BUDGET GUIDELINES

The objective of budgeting is to accurately forecast (on the basis of a set of assumptions) the volume of resources required to provide a specific mix and volume of services to patients over a defined period. In many hospitals, the budgeting process requires managers and directors to present their budget requests to their respective senior managers and the finance department. After this review, senior management and the finance team ask managers and directors to reduce their budget by a certain amount, making it clear that if the cuts are not deep enough the finance department will intervene to make the necessary adjustments.

This typical process puts the finance department in a negative light, earning this group the undeserved wrath of managers and directors. Such animosity can be prevented, however. Budgeting—a rite of passage for new managers, directors, and even vice presidents—should be collaborative, especially because it represents many initiatives geared toward a common cause: to provide appropriate care at a fair price and of the highest quality possible.

The energy expended on budget revisions can be minimized if clear guidelines are established and communicated to all budget participants at the start of the process. Budgeting guidelines should spell out the expectations and the parameters for the process, and they should be communicated before any budget work is done. This task is the responsibility of senior management. Guidelines must be supported by data—demographic, economic, and industry specific—from multiple sources. Demographic data aid in projecting future volumes; economic data are the basis for projecting inflation, interest rates, and overall economic growth; and industry data provide insights into new treatments and technologies. Data related to market share, profitability, past volumes, and possible rate adjustments should be trended.

After studying the data and the assumptions for the year, senior management can make projections and set parameters for expenses, patient volumes, test volumes, full-time equivalents (FTEs), and other key indicators. Budgets need to be established on the basis of data and assumptions that can be defended

with sound rationale. None of these data will be beneficial if senior management does not embrace the philosophy of transparency. When clear expectations are set and discussed ahead of time, a more realistic budget is created and supported by everyone involved in meeting it.

Without guidelines, managers and directors are more likely to request increases in their budgets. The net result may be an increase in expenses (including for FTEs) that are not based on current market conditions, resulting in a budget that the organization cannot justify. Again, sharing budgeting guidelines in advance saves a lot of work, minimizes frustration, and produces a better budget. See Figure 2.1 for three simple steps to improving the budgeting process.

A well-designed budget process is objective, preserves relationships,

Figure 2.1. Three Steps to a Better Budgeting Process

1. Review the organization's mission and strategic plan. These documents need to reflect the needs of the community.

2. Solicit input from stakeholders, including community representatives, employees, management, the medical staff, and the board of directors.

3. Establish and communicate clear budget guidelines. The guidelines should be based on industry benchmarks, changes in the environment, and the organization's past performance. Guidelines should be set for basic operating expenses, such as the number of FTEs per occupied bed or the number of FTEs per outpatient relative value unit.

supports the organization's values, and rewards performance. One of the best ways to reinforce desired behaviors, as well as values, is to publicly recognize individuals or departments that achieve their goals in a manner that supports the values.

Data are the basis for any budget, but an organization's values must always be the foundation for the budgeting process. That is to say, budget guidelines need to be applied fairly and consistently. Budgeting decisions based on favoritism, versus decisions based on objective data, undermine the budget and result in managers "gaming the system." (Consider the scenario in Sidebar G.) By avoiding favoritism or other unfair treatment in funding, the organization is reinforcing its values and strengthening its culture. For example, organizations should be consistent in how they approach joint ventures with members of the medical staff. Establishing a policy on joint ventures that is consistently followed eliminates the need to debate the issue each time it is presented.

Medical Staff Requests for Capital Purchases

A troubling financial issue that leaders learn to deal with is ad hoc requests made by members of the

SIDEBAR G

Hospital A's radiology department provides full service, including diagnostic radiology; MRI, CT, and PET scanning; and ultrasound. In the past three years, the total patient volume in the diagnostic radiology section has declined by 38 percent. The volume in the MRI section, on the other hand, has increased by 122 percent in the same time period. Three years ago, diagnostic radiology had its own supervisor, 14.5 FTEs, and a contribution margin of 64 percent, before indirect expense allocations. On the other hand, MRI shared its supervisor with the CT scanning section, had 6.2 FTEs, and had a contribution margin of 36 percent.

At the budget hearings this year, the supervisor for diagnostic radiology requested the same number of FTEs as required for last year, arguing that the section cannot cover the hours and provide the level of service expected by patients if the number of FTEs were reduced. However, MRI's contribution margin, before indirect allocations, has skyrocketed to 172 percent, compelling MRI's supervisor to request more staff. The radiology department, as a whole, cannot afford to budget for additional FTEs.

What can be done in this situation?

The radiology department must apply the established budget guidelines. Ideally, the manager or director of the department has been aware of the rise and fall of patient volumes in all sections of the unit and has been making the appropriate adjustments to the budget.

medical staff. Typically, such requests—ranging from approving a new program to purchasing new equipment—are brought to the CEO or another senior executive without having gone through the formal budgeting process.

In this scenario, a physician or group of physicians requests a meeting with the CEO. During the meeting, the physician makes a convincing case for his or her proposal, highlighting the competitive advantages, the additional revenues, the return on investment, and the service improvements that the project, program, or technology will bring. How can the CEO, acting on behalf of the organization, turn down such a great opportunity, particularly when it is endorsed by a valued member of the medical staff? The CEO needs to pause here.

Making capital financial decisions on an ad hoc basis not only eschews the budgeting process, but it will also be perceived as an act of favoritism that undermines the integrity of the process and the leader. Capital purchases or projects have to be evaluated on the basis of not just what the organization can afford but also what value they will provide to the community (Steuerle and Bovbjerg 2008). All hospitals need to have a capital budgeting process that is understood and followed fairly.

HOSPITAL SERVICES COMMITTEE. As mentioned, involving physicians in decision making is a major contributor to aligning their interests and values with those of the organization. One way to encourage physician involvement in strategy development, and in the capital budgeting process, is to form a committee that requires physician input in decision making. For our purposes, we will call this committee "hospital services committee," but the name is not im-

portant. This committee's purpose, structure, and functions have to be clearly articulated. By establishing this type of committee, the board and senior management are sending this message: We value and welcome the insights and participation of our medical staff in key decisions. When their opinions are sought, physicians are more apt to develop a sense of ownership of and commitment to the success of a project or capital purchase.

Also, if the medical staff believes that the decision-making process is fair and objective, they are more apt to be supportive, rather than contentious. Most importantly, formation of a hospital services committee is another way to reinforce a culture that values physician involvement. The financial benefits of participatory decision making are great, particularly when it comes to easing the increased competition and tension between hospitals and physicians (Burns, Anderson, and Shortell 1993).

Our proposed hospital services committee is a standing board committee. It should be structured as follows:

Purpose: To evaluate, and make a recommendation to the board of directors about, operating and capital budget requests from physicians that require board approval.

Functions:

- Solicit input from members of the medical staff related to operational issues and capital budgeting decisions that may have an impact on medical or clinical practice at the hospital. Broad physician participation ensures physician support for clinical-related projects.
- Create an objective decision-making process for capital purchases or projects. The objectivity of the process insulates the leader from charges of favoritism or having political motivations. Typically, the full board sets the criteria and dollar threshold for capital and operating decisions that require board approval. The committee ensures the process it has established follows the board criteria.
- Evaluate requests and proposals from various departments of the medical staff.
- Make recommendations to the full board or the finance committee of the board. The committee's recommendations are (or should be) tied directly to the organization's budget. Rejected proposals are most likely the result of the organization having limited resources relative to

the number of requests. Our experience suggests that requests that are denied in one year are often approved in the subsequent year.

Membership: The committee should be composed of six to eight members. The majority of members should be physicians who have active privileges at the hospital, and the rest should be made up of non-physicians who are senior managers or board members. The chairperson should be one of these three: (1) a physician who is an officer of the full board, (2) the chair of the medical executive committee (MEC), or (3) the vice chair of the MEC.

Capital requests must originate from the clinical department in which the sponsoring physician has privileges. This requirement ensures that the request is endorsed by a clinical department. A request that does not receive department approval is not forwarded to the hospital services committee. If a request is forwarded to the committee, the sponsoring physician is then asked to make a presentation to the committee.

All requests must include relevant financial and operational information, including direct and indirect expenses, additional staff, training requirements, modifications to the facility, and projected volumes and revenue based on the expected payer mix. The sponsoring physician must sign off on the projected volume information. This simple act of documenting projected volumes and signing the request helps to ensure that the projections are realistic. In our experience, sponsoring physicians do not make unrealistic projections because they know they will be held accountable for the results if the request goes through. That is, if the proposal is approved, the sponsoring physician must make a follow-up presentation to the board 6 to 12 months after the new program, service, or equipment has been installed.

Capital requests should be completed with assistance from the finance team. This request process is another way to encourage collaboration and teamwork between the finance staff and physicians.

RULE 6: SHARE INFORMATION AND HOLD PEOPLE ACCOUNTABLE

More organizations today are embracing the trend of transparency. Transparency allows everyone to be aware of what goals the organization is achieving (or not) and how their own roles contribute to organizational performance. Sharing information promotes a culture of trust and shared accountability.

Managers and directors are often reminded of the importance of meeting their financial goals. However, few organizations have formal mechanisms in place that hold managers and directors accountable for their budgets. Annual employee performance evaluations should be tied to financial objectives and specific organizational values. For example, a percentage of a manager's yearly raise should depend on whether he or she met, did not meet, or exceeded the budget. Similarly, if teamwork and innovation are two of the organization's values, they need to be incorporated into each employee's performance goals. At review time, each employee should be evaluated on how well he or she modeled these values and applied them to the work.

If employees—managers, directors, and line staff alike—are not held accountable for doing their part in following the budget, then two perceptions become realities:

1. Sticking to the budget is not important.
2. The CEO is solely responsible for achieving financial goals,

an impossible burden that contributes to a high rate of CEO turnover.

We cannot overemphasize the benefits of recognizing employees for excellent performance and for living the values of an organization. Recognition can be formal or informal, and it can be done privately or publicly; either way, sincere appreciation must be extended to the employee for a job well done.

RULE 7: UNCOVER THE HIDDEN EXPENSE OF TURNOVER

Ten years ago, few hospitals paid attention to staff turnover. Faced with cyclical nursing shortages, most hospitals did not investigate the reasons nurses were leaving; instead, they focused on recruiting more, a strategy that is analogous to bailing water out of a sinking ship instead of repairing the hole. Such recruitment efforts often resulted in bidding wars between hospitals, which perpetuated the issue and failed to address the underlying cause.

Enlightened hospitals, on the other hand, viewed the shortage as an opportunity. They evaluated the root causes—job dissatisfaction, low salary, shift scheduling, work overload, personal choices, and lack of continuing education, to name a few—and in the process, they were able to turn a negative into a positive. The following cases illustrate the cultural and financial benefits of low turnover.

Case 1. A hospital in the Midwest developed and implemented innovative programs designed to support employees and physicians. As a result, the hospital observed a remarkable reduction in turnover and vacancy rates. The hospital sustained this success by systematically listening to stakeholder concerns and continually responding to issues identified by employees and physicians. Low turnover, for this organization, translated into higher patient satisfaction, which generated increased market share, which funded programs and services that responded to the professional and personal needs of employees and the medical staff.

Case 2. SAS, a software company based in Cary, North Carolina, has a reputation for treating its employees well. In its 30 years of operation, SAS has never had a layoff, an impressive fact among many that was covered by a 2002 feature on the television show *60 Minutes* and in a 2007 article in *Fortune* magazine. At SAS, employee turnover has never exceeded 5 percent, another feat in an industry where the average turnover is 20 percent. As a result, "SAS saves $75 million a year in recruiting, training, and other turnover-related costs, while spending considerably less than $75 million on benefits" (Levering and Moskowitz 2007).

The successes in both of these cases are the direct result of an organization's culture that values not only its employees but also the judicious use of its financial resources.

RULE 8: DO NOT LOSE SIGHT OF THE MISSION, VISION, AND VALUES

The first step in the budgeting process should be to review the organization's mission to ensure that everyone understands why the organization exists. Virtually all healthcare organizations, regardless of their tax-exempt status, state that their mission is to provide needed healthcare services to their communities. The challenge for everyone is in keeping this focus on the mission and living the values, particularly in bad times.

Organizations that consistently adhere to their mission and values to reinforce their behaviors increase their chances of achieving sustainable success.

Our final thought on this last rule echoes the advice of healthcare futurist Leland Kaiser. Kaiser suggests that all not-for-profit hospitals should tithe or give 10 percent of their revenues to programs that respond to the specific needs of their communities. Services and initiatives selected for this funding should reflect the mission, vision, and values that shape the culture of the organization.

QUESTIONS FOR LEADERS

1. Why is a strong culture one of an organization's most important assets?
2. What strategies are effective in breaking down organizational silos or preventing them from developing?
3. Why is physician involvement important in developing and sustaining the culture of a healthcare organization?

4. Why should hospitals focus more on creating value for their communities than on growing their bottom lines?

5. How can budget guidelines help build a culture of teamwork?

6. Why is the mission statement an important document in budgeting?

REFERENCES

Altman, S. H., D. Shactman, and E. Eilat. 2006. "Could U.S. Hospitals Go the Way of U.S. Airlines?" *Health Affairs* 25 (1): 11–21.

American Management Association. 2002. "Communicating Up, Down, and Across the Organization: Influencing Your Stakeholders to Gain Support." Course Number W113. Chicago: American Management Association.

Berenson, R., P. Ginsburg, and J. May. 2006. "Hospital-Physician Relations: Cooperation, Competition, or Separation?" *Health Affairs* 26 (1): w31–43.

Burns, L. R., R. M. Anderson, and S. M. Shortell. 1993. "Trends in Hospital-Physician Relationships." *Health Affairs* 12 (3): 213–23.

Fisher, E. S., D. O. Staiger, J. Bynum, and D. J. Gottlieb. 2006. "Creating Accountable Care Organizations: The Extended Hospital Medical Staff." *Health Affairs* 26 (1): w44–57.

Healthcare Financial Management Association. 2007. *Key Hospital Financial Statistics and Ratio Medians.* Westchester, IL: HFMA.

Levering, R., and M. Moskowitz. 2007. "In Good Company." *Fortune* 155 (1): 94–96, 100.

McKinsey Quarterly. 2008. "The Link Between Management and Productivity." [Online information; retrieved 6/1/08.] www.mckinseyquarterly.com.

Nohria, N., W. Joyce, and B. Roberson. 2003. "What Really Works." *Harvard Business Review* 81 (7): 42–52.

Shortell, S. M., J. A. Alexander, P. P. Budetti, L. R. Burns, R. R. Gillies, T. M. Waters, and H. S. Zuckerman. 2001. "Physician-System Alignment: Introductory Overview." *Medical Care* 39 (7 Suppl 1): I1–8.

Steuerle, C. E., and R. R. Bovbjerg. 2008. "Health and Budget Reform as Handmaidens." *Health Affairs* 27 (3): 633–44.

CHAPTER 3

Leveraging Human Capital

> *People cannot be separated from their knowledge, skills, health, or values in the way they can be separated from their financial and physical assets.*
>
> —Gary S. Becker, Nobel Peace Prize–winning economist

Because healthcare is the business of people taking care of people, the concept of human capital is critical in this field. Simply stated, human capital is the collection of the contributions by employees that add value to the organization. This input, much of which is intangible such as caring, compassion, and loyalty, results in higher production, effectiveness, performance, and profit. Several schools of thought explain this concept, including those of labor economist Jacob Mincer and Nobel Peace Prize winner Gary Becker.

In this chapter, we discuss strategies that harness the power of human capital, the most important resource of any organization. ▶

PROVIDE ONGOING EDUCATION AND TRAINING

High-performing organizations understand the need to provide ongoing education and training to their employees. As mentioned in an article in *T+D Magazine* (2006, 30), "leaders who understand how to drive business results in an increasingly competitive environment recognize that a highly trained workforce improves performance."

According to a survey conducted by the American Society for Training and Development's (ASTD) Benchmarking Forum (BMF), a group of highly successful public and private companies, "the average annual expenditure per employee in BMF organizations increased to $1,424 per employee in 2005, an increase of 4.0 percent from 2004" (ASTD 2006, 3). The study also revealed a high trainer-to-employee ratio among this group. For example, Booz Allen Hamilton, ranked by ASTD as number one in promoting lifelong learning, boasts a trainer–employee ratio of 1:202. IBM is second on this list, with a ratio of 1:238.

Interestingly, no hospital or health system is included on this list. One possible reason for this is the way education and training are approached in the healthcare environment: Learning is presented in a one-size-fits-all medium, ignoring the needs and interests of the adult learner.

The Adult Learner

Andragogy is the study of how and why adults learn. Adult education expert Malcolm Knowles submits the three basic principles of andragogy (Atherton 2005):

1. Adults need to be involved in the planning and evaluation of their instruction.
2. Experience, including mistakes, provides the basis for learning activities.
3. Adults are most interested in learning about subjects that have immediate relevance to their job or personal life.

Often, these principles are not considered in the design and implementation of training in healthcare. For example, the CEO may determine that all staff will need to learn patient satisfaction approaches, leading to mandatory training. No one will argue that such an educational offering is beneficial and expands the values and culture of the organization. However, this or any other mandatory and elective training must be framed with the adult learner in mind to ensure that actual learning occurs. Learning can only occur if a person has the capacity (the how) and the motivation to learn (the why).

Converting learning into applied behavior requires a person's capacity, capability, and commitment. Tied to intelligence, capacity is a person's innate ability to understand and remember the material. Capability is the ability to use the information learned. Commitment, discussed later in the chapter, is the motivation to apply the learning.

A culture that values learning naturally nurtures a person's capacity, capability, and commitment. This workplace culture listens to the needs and wants of its employees and then responds with relevant, dynamic, and interactive learning opportunities.

Myths About Adult Learning

The commitment to pursue ongoing education and training is difficult to make for busy adults and for cash-strapped organizations. Compounding these factors are the mythology and misinformation about learning that have been hardwired into our collective mind-set. As a result, many organizations provide training that not only wastes limited resources but also fails to deliver its stated goals.

In this section, we challenge these myths and offer practical approaches to providing worthwhile education and training geared for adults. The basic truth in adult learning is that it should be self-directed and meaningful to the person involved.

MYTH 1: ADULTS LEARN BEST FROM EXPERTS WHO TELL THEM WHAT THEY NEED TO KNOW. Colleges and universities follow a rigorous curriculum designed to offer students as much academic experience and didactic knowledge as possible. Formal classroom learning, however, is neither practical nor appropriate for working people. Unfortunately, many healthcare organizations and professional associations apply this "university model" to their training initiatives for staff and physicians alike. They spend a great deal of time, money, and energy conducting needs-assessment surveys, holding focus groups, compiling data, and hiring consultants—all in an effort to create educational offerings that may be beneficial to their target audience.

Although the university model is suitable for a course in earning or maintaining professional credentials, or for a seminar related to culture building (e.g., a basic finance primer, as discussed in Chapter 2), it is impractical when applied to real-life scenarios and challenges. Working adults learn differently, and their training should relate to the work they perform, not what the experts deem to be important and current to their work and life.

MYTH 2: ADULTS LEARN BEST IN A PASSIVE LEARNING ENVIRONMENT. Interrelated with myth 1, this belief excludes the needs and wants of the learner. Many educational opportunities, such as board retreats, leadership development sessions, and management skill-building seminars, provide a platform for a "nationally renowned" guru to share his or her wisdom about a certain hot topic. Too often, these sessions turn into "edutainment," where the expert balances content with humor to make the participants feel good about attending. Whether actual learning occurs in these cases is questionable.

In many organizations, the method and length of time for education and training are dictated by the number of courses or hours of classroom instruction established by the department on the basis of the budget and continuing education requirements. For example, if the training department allotted funds for ten educational sessions for the year, and its performance review hinges on its delivery of (not the quality of) these ten sessions, then the department will make available ten sessions in a medium that is most feasible for the established budget. Often, the training method selected involves a lecture, not an interactive dialogue. Sadly, these input measures, rather than the desired outcomes, are often the primary focus of typical training programs.

As mentioned, adult learners relish the idea of being involved in and being able to relate to the educational experience they receive. Working adults are interested in participating and exchanging opinions, especially regarding topics that matter to their professional and personal life. Role playing, modeling, coaching, simulation, and mentoring are just some of the ways to stimulate adult learning.

Proactive Learning

The following are common techniques employed by high-performing healthcare organizations to facilitate participative learning:

- Listen to employees and the medical staff to gain insight into their education/training needs.

- Leverage the learner's strengths, not weaknesses. For example, a group of nurses would respond more positively to a training opportunity that teaches them how to develop clinical approaches. Conversely, they would begrudge a mandatory, and seemingly arbitrary, lesson in how to manage capital funds.
- Conduct "employee pride surveys" along with, or in place of, employee satisfaction surveys, to gather input on improving personal performance (see Atchison 1999; 2003). Healthcare organizations that attain sustainable success focus on employee pride first and employee satisfaction second. Pride is a visceral, long-term emotion, whereas satisfaction is a temporal, short-term feeling. While pride is the product of overcoming challenges, satisfaction is the result of an event that is pleasing. Pride is a deeper dimension that underpins high return on human capital (Atchison 2006).
- Focus on output, rather than input, measures. The goal or output of any educational program is to improve processes and performance. The training program should be measured in terms of how the learning was applied and what difference it made between the old and the new practices. Recording the number of training hours that each employee logs (an input) is a futile exercise because those hours do not ensure that the participants will use the knowledge to positively influence their future behavior.
- Engage and partner with learners to gain their commitment to education and training. Using contemporary learning methods, such as psychologist's Henry Mintzberg's (1994) strategic thinking processes, is one way to pursue this strategy.
- Reinforce lessons by providing opportunities that enable people (leaders, clinicians, and frontline employees) to apply what they learned. For example, if the training taught approaches for giving superior customer service, then a new procedure should be implemented that requires participants to be personally accountable for following up on any requests/orders, displaying positive behavior, and sharing relevant information.

An authority on organizational learning, professor Chris Argyris (1990; 2008) posits the "double-loop theory" when looking into adult learning. This idea is based on the premise that adults function with two mind-sets: (1) an "espoused theory"—what we say we do or believe in, and (2) a "theory-in-use"—what we actually do. Using double-loop theory allows us to evaluate the underlying reasons and background for the incongruence between what we say (perception) and what we do (reality). This system works for personal and professional pursuits. The alignment of words with behavior may be the most significant management characteristic required to maximize return on human capital. Employees watch management's behavior to determine whether these leaders are following their statements and promises with action. The fact is, no one is listening to what is said, but everybody is watching for what is done.

When applied to adult learning, double-loop theory enables the organization to understand that the major components of education are interaction and practice. Thus, surgeons cannot learn to operate by merely watching a surgical demonstration, administrators cannot learn to budget by just listening to a financial lecture, and nurse aides cannot learn to tend properly to a patient by simply attending a nursing class.

MEASURE HUMAN CAPITAL PERFORMANCE

To paraphrase the late management guru Peter Drucker, "information is data with meaning." Countless data exist in all healthcare organizations. Turning data into meaningful information is the work of both measurement and evaluation. Measurement refers to the systematic collection of data, while evaluation is the systematic interpretation of data. Accurate gathering and interpretation of data occur only when generally accepted methods are applied consistently. This statement is true for financial outcomes; it is also true for human capital performance.

In financial management, budgets, income statements, balance sheets, and ratio analyses are among the generally accepted methods for measuring and evaluating data. However, no such means are available for turning human capital data into information. Historically, the performance of the human resources has not been subjected to the rigorous and sophisticated methods applied to financial outcomes. The reason for this is that most organizations put much more emphasis on finance than on people. When people's performance does get measured and evaluated, the information is presented in a simplistic manner: "Our recent employee satisfaction scores put us at the 83rd percentile, which is 10 percentile points higher than last year's 73rd percentile. We are really doing great!" Imagine such a summarized report to the board about financial performance; that could end the career of an otherwise respected, competent leader.

Human capital must be managed as thoroughly as financial capital. That said, the approaches used for financial management can be applied to human capital management, including frequent monitoring and reporting, measurement and ratio scales, and even budgeting.

Frequent Monitoring and Reporting

Measurement and evaluation of human capital data are usually conducted annually, and sometimes every two years. This infrequency does not yield meaningful information on the return on investment in human capital. This practice needs to change. Human capital data must be collected, plotted, and analyzed with regularity. Most importantly, the results of this process must be shared with the board, management, employees, and physicians. See Table 3.1 for a grid comparing how human capital and financial capital are reported and monitored.

Most organizations rely on conducting employee opinion surveys

Table 3.1. Comparison of Reporting and Measurement for Financial Results and Human Capital Performance

	Financial Results	Human Capital Performance
Frequency	Often; some factors, daily	Yearly: major surveys (e.g., employee satisfaction)
Measurement scale	Ratio	Nominal, ordinal, and interval; occasionally ratio
Budgets	Detailed	Nonexistent
Board review	At every board meeting	As data are available or when problems surface

to gauge the collective attitude and perception of their staff. Although informative, the results of data collection performed only every other year may not be reliable because these responses may be dated and based on problems that existed long before the last survey. Certainly, more regular surveys can be carried out to get an accurate, current picture of the opinions of employees and physicians.

One alternative is to distribute a short (three to five questions) but specific questionnaire to a random sample of employees. These questionnaires can be designed to address specific departmental or organizational issues, such as turnover or quality. Presenting responses in a graphic format is an effective method of communicating survey data.

Another option is to hand out daily survey cards to targeted groups of employees. These cards may contain three to four statements that can be rated, from 5 (for strongly agree) to 1 (for strongly disagree); see Figure 3.1 for an example of this questionnaire. The time and location of distribution should vary every day to ensure even circulation throughout the facility and across all shifts. Also, questions on these cards should be different from day to day.

Figure 3.1. Pride Indicators

1 — Strongly Disagree	2 — Disagree	3 — Uncertain	4 — Agree	5 — Strongly Agree

_____ I have a sense of loyalty to this company.

_____ I identify with this company.

_____ I think about the future of this company.

_____ I've regretted that I chose to work for this company.

_____ I do extra work here because I want this company to succeed.

_____ I feel that I share in the success and failure of this company.

_____ I feel a sense of ownership in this company.

_____ It would take very little for me to move to another company.

_____ I take pride in being part of this company.

Shift: _____ Job Title: _____

Department: _____

Note: Please deposit your completed survey cards into the marked drop boxes throughout the hospital.

Source: Adapted with permission from Metritech, Inc. Champaign, Illinois.

Survey cards may be distributed every day for one month. Afterward, responses may be organized by shift, job title, length of service, and/or other variables that may have an impact on employee performance. Aggregate and unit-specific outcome data can be presented graphically to highlight trends and significant variations. Also, outcomes need to be reported to management and the human resources department, and a strategy should be in place to communicate these results to employees on a timely basis. Reporting results to employees as soon as possible is a surefire way to increase participation in future surveys as well as management's credibility.

Measurement Scales

Four basic scales can be used to measure human capital: nominal, ordinal, interval, and ratio.

Nominal scales group or organize data in categories, such as race, gender, and job title. *Ordinal scales* set the order of data, such as the most senior employee to the newest staff member, according to their value or their relationship with other data items. A Likert scale may be considered an ordinal scale in that it provides a series of ratings (e.g., strongly agree, neutral, strongly disagree) to questionnaire items.

Interval scales also rank order data but set presumably equal "intervals" between the ranking. With interval scales, each point supposedly represents the same value across the scale. A Fahrenheit temperature scale, for example, is an interval scale whereby each degree is equal. However, because interval scales use an arbitrary zero (the lowest point), the results are relative. For example, with a Fahrenheit scale, zero degree does not indicate a total lack of heat.

When using an interval scale, we can only speculate whether a rating of 4 is twice as good as a rating of 2, or if a score of 90th percentile is twice as high as 45th percentile.

Ratio scales function like interval scales, but these scales use an absolute zero. That is, four is twice as many as two, and a 240-pound patient weights twice as much as a 120-pound patient. With ratio scales, true comparisons across various groups can be made over time.

TIME AND BEHAVIOR. To collect, analyze, and present human capital data, preferred scales are nominal, ordinal, and interval. Ratio scales may be used to measure two human capital factors: time and behavior. Because a ratio scale has an absolute zero, it is appropriate for measuring common time indexes in hospitals, such as patient wait times in the emergency department, chart completion time, and hours of learning per full-time equivalent. A ratio scale may be used to effectively measure the following components related to employee behavior:

- Percentage of payroll invested in lifelong learning
- Turnover rate, segmented by age, discipline, and work unit

- Internal employee transfers, based on referrals by existing employees
- External hires, based on referrals by existing employees
- Quality patient care indicators (see Sidebar H)
- Attendance, including absenteeism

Behaviors are observable, repeatable, and measurable. These three straightforward traits indicate whether you are dealing with behavior or some other dynamic.

ATTITUDE AND EMOTION. Short surveys that are administered frequently and randomly yield insights into employee attitudes. Attitudes are personal opinions that can be influenced by an episode or event. For example, a nurse's attitude about the workload may change depending on the fluctuation of patient census on the floor. If volume is low today, the nurse's attitude may be positive. If demand is high tomorrow, then the nurse's outlook may be negative.

Likert scales are often used to measure attitude because they document a change in direction. Data gathered using Likert scales can be compared from period to period, allowing leaders to determine whether the numbers are rising, staying stable, or falling off the charts. The

SIDEBAR H

In 1999, the Institute of Medicine issued *To Err Is Human*, a publication reporting that up to 99,000 patients die each year in U.S. hospitals as a result of medical errors. This report challenged all healthcare professionals, including administrators and physicians, to deliver quality, timely clinical care 100 percent of the time.

The 100,000 Lives Campaign—a collaborative program initiated by Donald Berwick and the Institute for Healthcare Improvement (IHI) to save at least 100,000 lives per year with innovative interventions for preventing medical errors—has provided concrete evidence that measuring clinical outcomes improves patient care. The success of this program led to the 2006 launch of the 5 Million Lives Campaign, an extension of the original initiative. Almost two years into the program, the campaign is still going strong. According to IHI's *Fall Harvest* newsletter (see www.ihi.org), two of the multiple success factors documented by healthcare organizations that participate in the program are (1) regular monitoring and measurement of performance data and (2) investment in human capital and continuous learning.

simple format of a Likert scale eases the administration of the survey and the presentation of results.

Emotions, on the other hand, are deep feelings anchored in an individual's value system. Unlike attitudes, which are temporal and highly mutable, emotions are visceral and difficult to change. For example, a caregiver's strong religious beliefs may affect his or her feelings about medical scenarios that have sociopolitical undertones, such as abortion and euthanasia. Although none of the four scales discussed is useful in discerning emotion, a carefully designed scale may work to identify personal values.

As emphasized in this book, the strength of an organization's culture is determined by the level of values alignment between individual staff/ physicians/other caregivers and the institution itself. Most irreconcilable problems that occur on the job result when values are not clearly communicated and aligned. Figure 3.2 is an example of a values-based process to determine alignment of values.

VIEW HUMAN CAPITAL AS AN ASSET, NOT AN EXPENSE

When asked about how things are going, healthcare executives typically respond in the context of finance— whether performance is above or below budget. These same leaders seldom report on the condition of the organization's human capital. In fact, our experience is that most human resource issues are reactions to events, such as when union activity is on the horizon.

Low turnover, great employee pride, high productivity, and solid financial performance are just some of the benefits of tending to the needs of people. As such, human capital must be viewed as an investment, not an expense. This perspective not only encourages strategies and action that maximize the returns on this investment, but it also dispels the misconception that human capital is just another resource that costs money.

Chief People Officer

One strategy to change the mind-set about human capital is to create a position—which may be titled as chief people officer (CPO)—that serves as the head of all human capital activities and functions, including the human resources department. The CPO is responsible for leading the human capital budgeting process and for identifying and ensuring the use of appropriate metrics and reporting methodologies, much in the

---

Figure 3.2. Thematic Analysis (TA) Process and Steps

Definition: TA is an organizational development technique designed to use the personal experience of staff as the locus of change. The process maximizes involvement and motivation.

Steps

1. Silently write the "best" and "worst" personal experiences about any value (e.g., service, pride, communication).
2. In small groups (e.g., 6–8), have a round-robin discussion of "best" stories first.
3. After all of the best stories have been presented, discuss and select the most common themes in each story.
4. Use the most common themes to draft a "Standards for Performance" narrative for the value discussed.
5. Agree on a "standard," and then identify the current barriers to making the standard a reality.
6. Discuss all of the "worst" stories.
7. Identify the five worst themes.
8. Discuss if and when any of these negative behaviors are displayed.
9. Discuss ways to eliminate all negative themes.

way the chief financial officer (CFO) is charged with all finance functions. Having the CPO report directly to the CEO sends a message that people performance is just as important as financial performance.

Because installing a CPO, let alone treating the position as equal to a CFO, goes against the standard operating procedures of any healthcare organization, the success of this effort requires the full support of the CEO and the board of trustees. Support must go beyond mere lip service. Senior management and governance must regularly reinforce the benefits of having a CPO. Employees can determine the level of support for the CPO and for staff development when they see the amount of funding given to these elements, particularly when compared to other budget priorities.

FOSTER COMMITMENT

Commitment is an essential prerequisite for sustaining and improving returns on both human and financial capital. Senior management's commitment to the organization's culture and values motivates employees and physicians to support the mission and strategies of the enterprise. For example, at one hospital where

senior management's commitment was evident to everyone, a group of employees came forward with a request to start a hospital choir. This employee effort was a gesture of staff's commitment to the organization and its vision and culture.

Pride, loyalty, and ownership are the three major ingredients in commitment. With the understanding that engendering commitment is easier done within a strong culture, high-performing organizations, such as St. Luke's Health System in Idaho and St. Francis Hospital and Medical Center in Connecticut, invest time and resources to teach their managers and supervisors to foster a culture that values commitment. See Figure 3.3 for strategies that follow the example of successful organizations.

Pride

Pride is the feeling of accomplishment, especially in the face of a challenging task. Pride is akin to happiness and satisfaction. However, satisfaction is temporal, while pride is visceral.

Feeling proud of the work done is not just about completing the task at hand. The task itself has to be meaningful and must be within the person's capability (Atchison 2006, 33). Different from the temporary sensation of satisfaction, pride is long

Figure 3.3. Strategies for Building Commitment

1. Develop an inspiring vision, and foster team commitment to it.
2. Create a listening environment.
3. Recognize and reward teamwork among those who help the team.
4. Implement team projects.
5. Recruit qualified people who are enthusiastic about team participation.
6. Ensure that all professional development necessary for members of a team to function successfully is made available to them.
7. Ensure that support systems are in place.
8. Promote and encourage change, innovation, and risk taking.
9. Communicate the results of team efforts across the organization.
10. Remind staff that they will either win as a team or lose as a team.
11. Build a strong team and then give its members credit for their efforts.
12. Celebrate *all* successes.

lasting because achieving it demands more, including energy, concentration, intellectual skill, and maturity. People who are proud of their work tend to share their success stories with others, which can be inspiring. For more information about pride, see Atchison (2003; 2006).

Loyalty

Simply, loyalty is devotion. In the workplace, loyalty is a person's willingness to stick with an organization through good and bad times. The unrelenting changes in the healthcare industry make loyalty to the organization a rare commodity.

Following are some truths about loyalty in the healthcare workplace:

1. *Not everyone should be loyal.* Let's face it, not all employees are star performers. To maximize the return on human capital, star performers must be frequently rewarded, separating them from the low performers and possibly encouraging better work from everybody else. Ideally, all employees are highly capable and have individual values that are aligned with those of the organization. Realistically, however, many staff members are not a good match in capacity or values. Therefore, leaders and managers should not enable and want loyalty from those who are less-than-satisfactory workers and whose behavior disrupts the established culture.

2. *Employees tend to be more loyal to their boss and peers than to their organization.* Human resource executives have long known that turnover is linked to poor supervision; the relationship between an employee and his or her direct supervisor is the biggest determinant in this equation. In light of this fact, engendering loyalty must start with training

supervisors in selecting, motivating, and rewarding employees.

3. *Physicians are loyal to their patients, not to the organization.* The primary focus of physicians who practice and are credentialed in any hospital is to meet the medical needs of their patients. If the organization seeks physician loyalty, the organization must "make it easy for physicians to practice," must be adaptable to changes, and must deliver high-quality care (Teska and Wolosin 2006). This means that leaders must ensure that the institution allows physicians to provide modern, efficient care that strengthens and adds value to everyone's reputation within the community. Physicians who are proud to be affiliated with such an organization bring in referral business.

Ownership

Ownership is the outcome of open communication and engagement. Before and after a change occurs, successful leaders communicate with all stakeholders in the organization. They discuss what is currently going on, what will happen in the future, why the change is necessary, and how the change will affect everyone involved.

For some people, open communication alone is a clear indication of the organization's willingness to be inclusive. But successful leaders go a step beyond: They engage everyone as well, welcoming ideas, questions, and recommendations. A combination of these two processes fosters ownership, a feeling that one is part of the big picture. The more that employees and physicians believe that they have a voice in decision making, the greater their sense of ownership.

QUESTIONS FOR LEADERS

1. Does your organization have a lifelong education program that seeks input from and considers the development needs of staff and physicians?

2. Are your professional development courses focused primarily on teaching practical solutions to immediate situations?

3. Do you measure the performance of your human capital? How do you measure time, behavior, attitudes, and emotions?

4. How do you view your human capital? Does it get less attention than your financial resources?

5. What specific processes do you have in place to build commitment? How do you measure pride, loyalty, and ownership?

REFERENCES

American Society for Training and Development (ASTD). 2006. "ASTD Research Update." [Online information; retrieved 6/1/08.] http://astd2007.astd.org/PDFs/Handouts%20for%20Web/Handouts%20Secured%20for%20Web%205-17%20thru%205-22/TU204.pdf.

Argyris. C. 2008. *Teaching Smart People How to Learn*. Boston: Harvard Business School Press.

———. 1990. *Overcoming Organizational Defenses: Facilitating Organizational Learning*. New York: Prentice Hall.

Atchison, T. 2006. *Leadership's Deeper Dimensions*. Chicago: Health Administration Press.

———. 2003. "Exposing the Myths of Employee Satisfaction." *Healthcare Executive* 18 (3): 20–26.

———. 1999. "The Myths of Employee Satisfaction." *Healthcare Executive* 14 (2): 18–23.

Atherton, J. S. 2005. "Learning and Teaching: Knowles' Andragogy: An Angle on Adult Learning." *T+D Magazine*.

Becker, G. undated. "Human Capital." [Online article; retrieved 9/3/08.] www.econlib.org/library/Enc/HumanCapital.html.

Institute of Medicine. 1999. *To Err Is Human*. Washington, DC: National Academies Press.

Mintzberg, H. 1994. *Rise and Fall of Strategic Planning*. New York: Free Press.

T+D Magazine. 2006. "Investing in Learning; Looking for Performance." *T+D Magazine*, p. 30.

Teska, L., and R. Wolosin. 2006. "A More Heartfelt Loyalty." [Online article; retrieved 6/1/08.] www.hhnmag.com/hhnmag_app/hospitalconnect/search/article.jsp?dcrpath = HHNMAG/PubsNewsArticle/data/2006April/060404HHN_Online_Teska&domain = HHNMAG.

SUGGESTED READING LIST

American Society for Training and Development. 2006. "ASTD Research Update." www.astd.org.

Argyris. C. 1990. *Overcoming Organizational Defenses: Facilitating Organizational Learning.* New York: Prentice Hall.

———. 2008. *Teaching Smart People How to Learn.* Boston: Harvard Business School Press.

Atchison, T. 2003. *Followership.* Chicago: Health Administration Press.

———. 2003. "Exposing the Myths of Employee Satisfaction." *Healthcare Executive* 18 (3): 20–26.

———. 2006. *Leadership's Deeper Dimensions.* Chicago: Health Administration Press.

Atherton, J. S. 2005. "Learning and Teaching: Knowles' Andragogy: An Angle on Adult Learning." *T+D Magazine.*

Becker, G. undated. "Human Capital." www.econlib.org/library/Enc/HumanCapital.html.

Berenson, R., P. Ginsburg, and J. May. 2006. "Hospital–Physician Relations: Cooperation, Competition, or Separation." *Health Affairs* 26 (1): w31–43.

Cummings, T. G., and C. G. Worley. 2004. *Organization Development and Change,* 8th ed. Florence, KY: South-Western College Publishing.

Fisher, E. S., D. O. Staiger, J. Bynum, and D. J. Gottlieb. 2006. "Creating Accountable Care Organizations: The Extended Hospital Medical Staff." *Health Affairs* 26 (1): w44–57.

Healthcare Financial Management Association. 2007. *Key Hospital Financial Statistics and Ratio Medians.* Westchester, IL: HFMA.

Heathfield, S. 2008. "How to Change Your Culture: Organizational Culture Change." www.about.com.

Herzberg, F. 2003. "One More Time: How Do You Motivate Employees?" *Harvard Business Review* 81 (1): 87–96.

Levering, R., and M. Moskowitz. 2007. "In Good Company." *Fortune* 155 (1): 94–96, 100.

McKinsey Quarterly. 2008. "The Link Between Management and Productivity." www.mckinseyquarterly.com.

Nohria, N., W. Joyce, and B. Roberson. 2003. "What Really Works." *Harvard Business Review* 81 (7): 42–52.

Steuerle, C. E., and R. R. Bovbjerg. 2008. "Health and Budget Reform as Handmaidens." *Health Affairs* 27 (3): 633–44.

T+D Magazine. 2006. "Investing in Learning; Looking for Performance." *T+D Magazine,* p. 30.

Teska, L., and R. Wolosin. 2006. "A More Heartfelt Loyalty." www.hhnmag.com.

ABOUT THE AUTHORS

Tom Atchison, EdD, is president and founder of The Atchison Consulting Group, Inc. Since 1984, Dr. Atchison has consulted with healthcare organizations on managed-change programs, teambuilding, and leadership development. He also has consulted to the military, healthcare vendors, and government agencies on the intangible aspects of healthcare. His consulting practice focuses on measuring and managing the intangibles that drive change. Typically, he consults to senior executives, managers, trustees, and physician leaders.

Dr. Atchison presents to thousands of healthcare professionals every year on the elements of effective organizations. He has written and been featured in a number of articles, audiotapes, and videotapes about motivation, managed change, teambuilding, and leadership. He is the author of four books: *Turning Healthcare Leadership Around, Leading Transformational Change: The Physician–Executive Partnership, Followership: A Practical Guide to Aligning Leaders and Followers,* and *Leadership's Deeper Dimensions: Building Blocks to Superior Performance.*

Dr. Atchison's expertise in healthcare is built on more than 30 years of experience in a variety of management positions in healthcare institu-tions and organizations. An affiliate of the American College of Healthcare Executives, he earned a doctorate in human resource development from Loyola University Chicago.

Greg Carlson, PhD, is manager of Global Health Services at Kimberly-Clark Corporation and serves as an adjunct faculty member at the University of South Carolina and at Georgia State University. For ten years, he was chief executive officer of a 500-bed freestanding healthcare system with more than 2,500 employees.

As a hospital CEO, Dr. Carlson led earnings growth, implemented four rate reductions, introduced a hospitalwide quality-monitoring system, reduced employee turnover by 50 percent, and increased internal promotions by more than 60 percent. He was instrumental in merging two hospitals and creating an award-winning wellness facility described as a "hospital without beds," focused on education, community wellness, prevention, and outpatient services.

Dr. Carlson serves as chairman of the board of directors of PE 4 Life, an advocacy group working to address childhood obesity in our schools. He earned a master's in health administration from the University of Pittsburgh and a doctorate in health policy from the University of South Carolina.

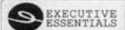
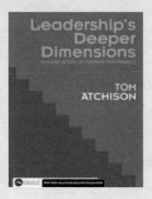

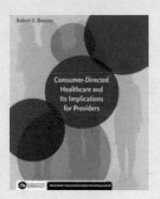

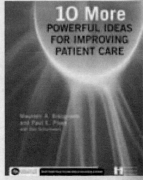

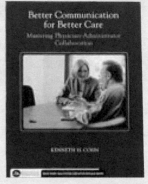

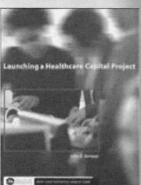

Straightforward

Executive Essentials books have a straightforward layout. Information is easy to read and find.

Focused

Executive Essentials books provide the most vital information on a topic. You won't get bogged down in superfluous details. If you do want to dig deeper into the subject, we provide a list of additional resources.

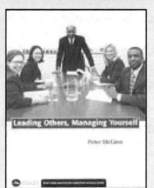

Practical

Executive Essentials books provide ready-to-use forms, charts, and checklists. Organize your work with these helpful tools.

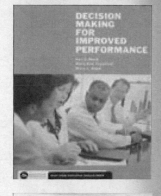

Concise

Executive Essentials books get right to the point. Each book is 80 pages or less.

Portable

Executive Essentials books are light enough to travel with you. Learn valuable information while flying or commuting.

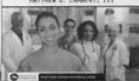